Health Fitness Activities

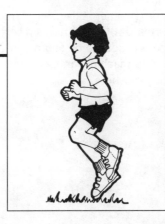

by Janet A. Wessel and Ellen Curtis-Pierce

Fearon Teacher Aids
Belmont, California

Designed and Illustrated by Rose C. Sheifer

ISBN 0-8224-5353-3

Printed in the United States of America

1. 9 8 7 6 5 4 3 2 1

Contents

Meeting Special Needs of Children

AIMS OF THE PROGRAM

In any class, one or more students may be unable to play and perform basic motor skills effectively. If these students can't play, run, jump, and throw at an early age, they may be slow to develop essential motor skills as well as other basic learnings and social skills—or not develop them at all.

Play is a child's way of learning and integrating skills that will be used throughout life. Through play, children come to understand the world about them. Through play, children learn to move and move to learn. And as children gain play and motor skills, their feelings of self-worth and their positive self-images grow.

Most children learn to play and move through the activities of childhood. They learn by interacting with the environment and with their brothers and sisters and their peers. Handicapped children and other children with special needs often lack the opportunities to play with their peers. These children do not develop play and motor skills on their own. They need a structured, sequential curriculum to interact with their peers, gain feelings of self-worth, and achieve success—and the sooner these children can begin such a program, the better.

This Play and Motor Skills Activities Series presents a program of effective instruction strategies through which all children can achieve success in the general physical education program. It is not a pull-out program (that is, the child is not pulled out for therapy or special tutorial assistance); it is not a fix-it program (that is, the child is not segregated until all deficits are remediated). It is a positive program for each child to succeed in a play-and-motor-skills activity program. It is designed to help you, the teacher, set up sequential curricula, plan each child's instructional program, and teach effectively so that each child progresses toward desired learning outcomes.

Three Major Aims of the Program

1. To enable each child to perform basic play and motor skills at the level of his or her abilities;

2. To help each child use these skills in play and daily living activities to maximize his or her health, growth, and development, as well as joy in movement; and

3. To enhance each child's feelings of self-worth and self-confidence as a learner while moving to learn and learning to move.

BOOKS IN THE SERIES

There are eight books in this Play and Motor Skills Activities Series for preprimary through early primary grades, ages 3–7 years.

1. Locomotor Activities
2. Ball-Handling Activities
3. Stunts and Tumbling Activities
4. Health and Fitness Activities
5. Rhythmic Activities
6. Body Management Activities
7. Play Activities
8. Planning for Teaching

The seven activities books are designed to help teachers of children with handicaps and other special-needs children. Each book provides sequential curricula by skill levels. Each book is complete within its cover: sequential skills and teaching activities, games, action words, and checklists for the class's record of progress in each skill and an Individual Record of Progress (IRP) report.

Book 8, *Planning for Teaching*, is an essential companion to each of the seven activities books because it presents not only the steps for planning a teaching unit and providing for individual differences in each lesson, but it also includes a guide to incorporating social skills into units and lessons and also outlines a Home Activities Program. These two guides are particularly important for children with special needs. Because they often have limited opportunities to interact with their peers, these children need planned, sequential learning experiences to develop socially acceptable behaviors. And because special-needs children also often need extensive practice to retain a skill and generalize its use, a Home Activities Program, planned jointly by parents and teacher, can give them the necessary additional structured learning opportunities.

SEQUENTIAL CURRICULA: SUCCESS BY LEVELS

Each child and the teacher evaluate success. Success is built into the sequential curricula by levels of skills and teaching activities.

Each skill is divided into three levels: rudimentary Skill Level 1 and more refined Skill Levels 2 and 3. Each level is stated in observable behavioral movement terms. The skill levels become performance objectives. Children enter the sequential program at their own performance levels. As they add one small success to another and gain a new skill component or move to a higher skill level, they learn to listen, follow directions, practice, create, and play with others.

Within each skill level, your activities are sequenced, so the child can gain understanding progressively. Within each skill, you provide cues to meet each child's level of understanding and ability. The continuum of teaching cues is

1. verbal cues (action words) with physical assistance or prompts throughout the movement,

2. verbal cues and demonstrations,

3. verbal challenges and problem-solving cues such as "can you?" and

4. introduction of self-initiated learning activities.

GAMES

Game activities are identified for each performance objective by skill level in the seven activity books. At the end of each activity book is an alphabetized description of the games. This list includes the name of each game, formation, directions, equipment, skills involved in playing, and the type of play. Just before the list, you'll find selection criteria and ways to adapt games to different skill levels. Many of the game activities can be used to teach several objectives.

ACTION WORDS

Words for actions (step, look, catch, kick), objects (foot, ball, hand), and concepts (slow, fast, far) are used as verbal cues in teaching. These action words should be matched to the child's level of understanding. They provide a bridge to connect skill activities with other classroom learnings. In the seven activity books, action words are identified for each performance objective by skill level, and an alphabetized list of Action Words is provided at the beginning of each book. As you use this program, add words that are used in other classroom activities and delete those that the children are not ready to understand.

CHECKLISTS: A CHILD'S RECORD OF PROGRESS

In each activity book, you'll also find Individual and Class Records of Progress listing each performance objective. You can use one or both to record the entry performance level and progress of each child. The child's Individual Record of Progress can be used as part of the Individualized Educational Program (IEP). The teacher can record the child's entry performance level and progress on the child's IEP report form or use the end-of-the-year checklist report.

By observing each child performing the skills in class (e.g., during play, during teaching of the skill or in set-aside time), you can meet the special needs of each child. By using the checklists to record each child's entry level performance of objectives to be taught, you can develop an instructional plan for and evaluate the progress of each child.

Assign each child a learning task (skill component or skill level) based on lesson objectives, and plan lesson activities based on the entry performance level to help the child achieve success. Then use the checklists to record, evaluate, and report each child's progress to the parents. With this record of progress, you can review the teaching-learning activities and can make changes to improve them as necessary.

TEACHING STRATEGY

Direct Instruction

Direct Instruction is coaching on specific tasks at a skill level that allows each child to succeed. A structured and sequential curriculum of essential skills is the primary component of Direct Instruction. As the child progresses in learning, the teacher poses verbal challenges and problem-solving questions such as "can you?" and "show me!" Direct Instruction is based on the premise that success builds success and failure breeds failure.

Adaptive Instruction

Adaptive Instruction is modifying what is taught and how it is taught in order to respond to each child's special needs. Adaptive Instruction helps teachers become more responsive to individual needs. Teaching is based on the child's abilities, on what is to be taught in the lesson, and on what the child is to achieve at the end of instruction. Lesson plans are based on the child's entry performance level on the skills to be taught. Students are monitored during instruction, and the activities are adjusted to each student's needs. Positive reinforcement is provided, and ways to correct the performance or behavior are immediately demonstrated.

Children enter the curriculum at different skill levels, and they learn at different rates. The sequential curriculum helps teachers to individualize the instruction for each child in the class. Thus, the same skill can be taught in a class that includes Betty, who enters at Skill Level 1, and James, who enters at Skill Level 3, because the activities are prescribed for the class or group, but the lesson is planned in order to focus on each child's learning task, and each child is working to achieve his or her own learning task. What is important is that each child master the essential skills at a level of performance that matches his or her abilities, interests, and joy.

Since children learn skills at different rates, you might want to use the following time estimates to allot instructional time for a child to make meaningful progress toward the desired level of performance. One or two skill components can usually be mastered in the instructional time available.

120 minutes	180 minutes	240 minutes	360 minutes
▲	▲	▲	▲

Higher Functioning Faster Learner   Slower Functioning Slower Learner

Health Fitness Skills and Activities

INTRODUCTION

Goals for Each Child

1. To demonstrate the ability to perform health fitness skills taught in the instructional program;

2. To use health fitness skills in daily living activities in order to maximize healthy development and joy in movement; and

3. To gain greater feelings of self-worth and self-confidence and to gain greater ability in moving to learn and learning to move.

Physical fitness is important to healthy well-being. It is an integral part of the play and motor skills program for children with special needs. The development of optimal levels of physical fitness as a child grows and matures is a major program goal.

The key elements of physical fitness are (1) endurance and stamina, or the well-being of the heart, lungs, and blood vessels; (2) muscular strength, capacity for movement, and prevention of injury; and (3) flexibility, or the optimal range of motion of body joints.

Fitness also includes rest and relaxation, or the ability to release muscular tension; good posture and the prevention of back injury through appropriate body alignment in lifting and carrying weights; and weight control appropriate for the individual's nutrition and physical activity.

Physical fitness is developed and maintained through appropriate amounts and types of physical activities at home and in school, which include the following:

1. *For endurance and stamina:* large muscle activities such as walking, running, skipping, galloping, biking, swimming, and selected rhythmic activities involving locomotor skills (these activities are also important for weight control);

2. *For muscular strength:* movement activities such as creeping, crawling, climbing, jumping, and specific strength exercises for the abdominal, back, leg, and arm-chest-shoulder muscles;

3. *For flexibility:* movement activities such as bending, turning, twisting, and reaching, and exercises for specific joints;

4. *For lifting and carrying objects:* movement activities involving appropriate body alignment and using the large leg muscles to do the lifting, thus preventing back injury;

5. *For rest and relaxation:* movement activities to release muscular tension in various parts of the body and in the total body.

Incorporating this entire range of physical fitness activities into the program of play and motor skills activities is essential; it doesn't matter which of the specific exercise movements listed you use.

Many children with special needs lack the skills or opportunities to participate in physical fitness activities. Not only does this lead to low levels of physical fitness, but it also leads to difficulty in acquiring play and motor skills. Physical fitness is essential to many play and motor skills.

This book presents activities by three skill levels for each of the physical fitness elements in the following order:

1. Situps (abdominal strength)
2. Walk-run (heart-lung endurance and stamina)
3. Trunk and leg flexibility
4. Lifting and carrying objects (posture)
5. Rest and relaxation

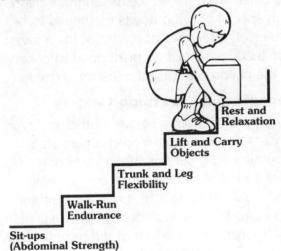

Rest and Relaxation
Lift and Carry Objects
Trunk and Leg Flexibility
Walk-Run Endurance
Sit-ups (Abdominal Strength)

GETTING STARTED

To begin, decide which health fitness skills you will teach. You can plan a unit or a week or a day or a year. You may decide to teach all skills in this book. Or you may select just a few. Review the checklist for each skill objective you select to teach. Become familiar with the skill components. Next, decide which action words and games you will use in teaching these skills.

Action Words

The words you use are teaching cues. Select ones your children will understand. For each of the health fitness skills, action words are listed by skill level, and an alphabetized list of words for all the skills in this book is provided below. Circle the words you will use in teaching. If the words you selected prove too difficult for your students, cross them out. Add others that are more appropriate for your children. Star those words that work well.

ACTION	OBJECT	CONCEPT
Bend	Arm	Back
Breathing	Back	Backward
Carry	Bases	Both
Control	Bench	Close
Curl	Block	Down
Go	Box	Fast
Grasp	Chin	Feel
Hold	Cones	Flat
Lean	Drum	Forward
Lie	Eyes	Front
Lift	Face	Hard
Move	Fingers	Let go
Pick up	Fist	Look
Put down	Floor	Lower
Raise	Foot	Ready
Reach	Footprints	Relax
Return	Hand	Show me
Run	Head	Side
Sit	Knee	Slow
Squeeze tight	Leg	Slowly
Stand	Line	Start
Start	Mat	Straight
Step	Shoulder	Tense
Stop	Stick	Tight
Tuck	Tape	Up
Uncurl	Toe	Upper
Walk	Toy	
	Trunk	
	Yardstick	

Games and Play Activities

For each skill level, you'll find a list of games; select the activity matched to the skills you plan to teach. At the end of this book, you'll find a list of games along with a description of each of them. You'll note that some of the games can be used to teach more than one skill. Use this master list to note those games and play activities that work well and those that do not. Make your comments right on the game listed, or set up a similar format for the games you have selected and make your comments on that sheet. This kind of information can help you plan successful teaching activities.

Equipment

One or more of the following pieces of equipment will be needed for most of the health fitness activities and games:

1. Mats
2. Boxes of various weights (1–2 lbs.)
3. Traffic cones
4. Bases or carpet squares
5. Drum, tambourine
6. Box with rules (sit-and-reach bench)
7. Whistle for signals
8. Class name chart and star stickers
9. Colored tape to mark the floor to space equipment safely
10. Table
11. Balls of various sizes (nerf, 6" playground ball, medicine ball)
12. Water buckets and large plastic strip
13. Small toys—trucks, wagons, building blocks
14. Child-size footprints cut out or painted on boxes or benches.

Space

Health fitness activities require enough space for each child to move comfortably and safely. The size of the space depends on the equipment available for the activities and games selected and on the number of children in the class. A multipurpose room and a playground are desirable.

Health and Safety

Space and the equipment should be arranged for safety (mats for situps, leg flexibility, relaxation). Children with braces or crutches or special visual needs may need a tour of the space and equipment before the lesson. A buddy can be assigned to be near the child when the lesson is taught. Children with special hearing needs may need to be close to the teacher or leader of the activity. The teacher should be positioned to observe all the children during the lesson activities.

Organization: Learning Centers

Learning centers are one of the best types of class organization. You can plan small group learning centers when you know each child's level of performance of the health fitness skill to be taught. Learning centers can be used to group children by levels of ability or to mix children of different levels of ability. The number of learning centers and their purpose will depend on the number of teachers and support personnel: aides, parent volunteers, older peer models.

To set up a learning center, you should consider the following:

1. Purpose	Skills to be taught and practiced
2. Levels	Levels 1, 2, and 3, or only one, determined by size of class, space, equipment, support personnel
3. Grouping	Same or mixed skill levels
4. Physical setting	Location, such as playground or multipurpose room; equipment available; existing physical boundaries, such as walls, or space to make boundaries with chairs, benches, mats, tapes
5. Activities	Type of game or instructional activity, such as running on paths, jumping over lines, climbing jungle gym

LEARNING CENTERS: HEALTH FITNESS ACTIVITIES

LEARNING CENTER 1

Location: Playground

Skill: Situps, leg flexibility, walk-run for endurance

Activity: Perform situps, sit and reach, walk-run

Grouping: Children at same or different skill levels

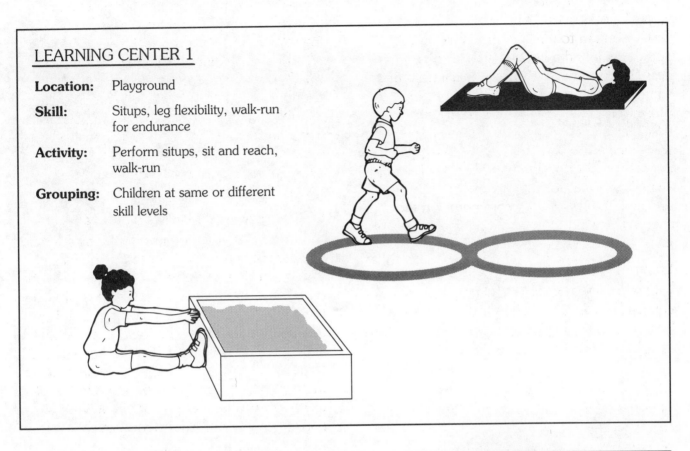

LEARNING CENTER 2

Location: Classroom

Skill: Lifting and carrying and relaxation

Activity: Lift and carry books, blocks into container, water to sink; relaxation on carpet

Grouping: Children at same or different skill levels

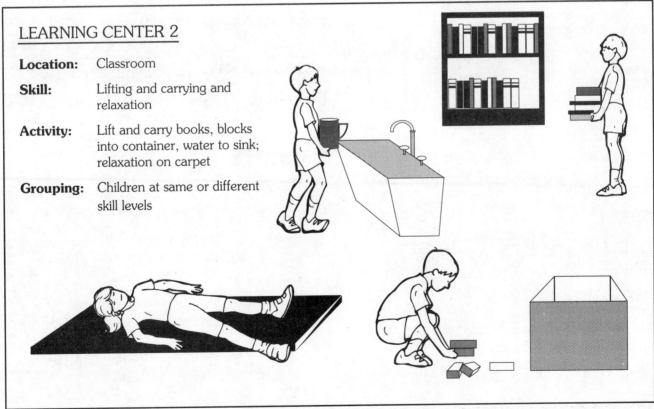

Health Fitness Activities

SITUPS (ABDOMINAL STRENGTH): SKILL LEVEL 1

Performance Objective

The child with ability to assume a ready position (legs bent, reclining) can perform a situp three consecutive times, demonstrating the following skill components:

On an 8-foot mat, the child can

1. take a starting position (lying on back, knees bent 90 degrees, feet flat on mat, arms at sides, feet supported), then

2. curl up by tucking chin and lifting shoulders (upper back) off the mat and

3. return to starting position in a controlled movement by uncurling and lowering head to mat.

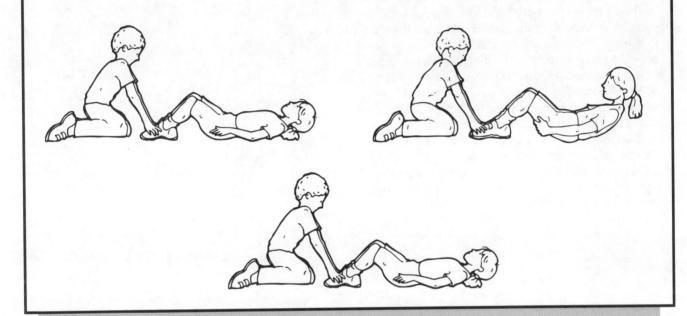

Action Words

Actions: Bend, control, curl, lie, lift, raise, return, sit, tuck, uncurl

Objects: Arm, back, chin, drum, foot, floor, hand, head, knee, mat, shoulder, toy

Concepts: Down, flat, look, ready, show me, up, upper

Games

- Beat the Stars
- Did You Ever See a Lassie/Laddie?
- Follow the Leader
- Obstacle Course
- Simon Says
- Trunk Lifts

TEACHING ACTIVITIES

If a child requires assistance to respond,

1. give verbal cues and physical assistance.
Manipulate or guide the child onto back with legs bent. Have a partner hold ankles. Place the child's arms at sides. Lift the child's head, shoulders, and upper back off the floor. Return slowly to mat. Give the child specific verbal instructions throughout (in sign language, bliss symbols, action cues), such as "Sit up," "Lie down."

2. give verbal cues with demonstration.
Use a model or have the child watch you raise your head, shoulders, and upper back off the floor while assuming a bent-leg, reclining position. Then have the child perform the action. Use specific verbal instructions (as in 1 above with the modeling).

If a child can respond without assistance,

3. **give a verbal challenge in the form of a problem: "Who can . . . ?" "Show me how you can . . ."**

   a. Ring the bell held above your knees as you raise yourself up.

   b. Grab the toy on your knees as you raise yourself up.

   c. Touch your knees as you raise yourself up.

   d. Variation: Raise up to beat of drum.

4. **introduce self-initiated learning activities.** Set up the mats and space for situps. Provide time at the beginning of the lesson and free time for independent learning after the child understands the skills to be used. You may ask the child to create a game activity to play alone or with others (partner or small group) on carpet squares or mats.

5. **Variations:** Set up an obstacle course that includes colored tape and mats to perform situps. Play a game, such as Follow the Leader, Simon Says, or Beat the Stars, that incorporates situp activities. Health fitness activities such as walking, running, rolling, climbing, creeping, and crawling are also important movements in developing and maintaining strength in the abdominal and back muscles.

SITUPS (ABDOMINAL STRENGTH): SKILL LEVEL 2

Performance Objective

The child with acquisition of Skill Level 1 can perform a situp three consecutive times, demonstrating the following skill components:

On an 8-foot mat, the child can

4. curl up by tucking chin and lifting trunk, complete the curl by touching the knees with hands, and

5. return in a controlled manner by uncurling trunk and lowering head to mat, hands on thighs, and then

6. repeat ten times (or meet standards that are appropriate for the child).

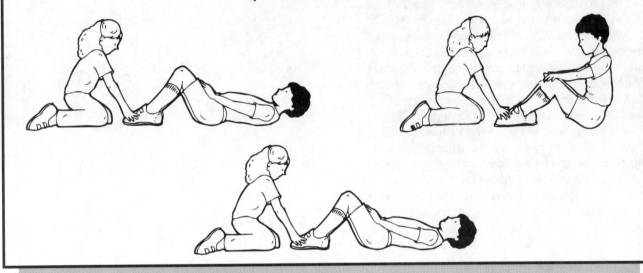

Skills to Review

1. Take a starting position (lying on back, knees bent 90 degrees, feet flat on mat, arms at sides, feet supported), then

2. curl up by tucking chin and lifting shoulders (upper back) off the mat and

3. return to starting position in controlled movement by uncurling and lowering head to mat.

Action Words

Actions: Bend, control, curl, lie, lift, raise, return, sit, tuck, uncurl

Objects: Arm, back, chin, drum, foot, floor, hands, head, knee, mat, shoulder, toy

Concepts: Down, flat, look, ready, show me, up, upper

Games

- Beat the Stars
- Did You Ever See a Lassie/Laddie?
- Follow the Leader
- Obstacle Course
- Simon Says
- Trunk Lifts

TEACHING ACTIVITIES

If a child requires assistance to respond,

1. give verbal cues and physical assistance.
Manipulate or guide the child onto back with legs bent. Have a partner hold ankles. Place the child's arms at sides. Lift the child's head and trunk off the floor to a sitting position so that arms can touch knees. Return slowly to floor. Give the child specific verbal instructions throughout (in sign language, bliss symbols, action cues), such as "Sit up," "Lie down."

2. give verbal cues with demonstration.
Use a model or have the child watch you raise your head and trunk off the floor to a sitting position with arms touching knees and return to floor. Repeat. Then have the child perform the action. Use specific verbal instructions (as in 1 above with the modeling).

If a child can respond without assistance,

3. give a verbal challenge in the form of a problem: "Who can . . . ?" "Show me how you can . . ."

a. Grab the toy by your ankles as you sit up and bring it to your chest.

b. Hit your knees with your hand every time you curl up.

c. Count the number of situps you can do in one time period (teacher sets time).

d. Variation: Do situps to beat of drum.

4. introduce self-initiated learning activities. Set up the mats and space for situps. Provide time at the beginning of the lesson and free time for independent learning after the child understands the skills to be used. You may ask the child to create a game activity to play alone or with others (partner or small group) on carpet squares or mats.

5. Variations: Set up an obstacle course that includes colored tape and mats to perform situps. Play a game, such as Follow the Leader, Simon Says, or Beat the Stars, that incorporates situp activities. Health fitness activities such as walking, running, rolling, climbing, creeping, and crawling are also important movements in developing and maintaining strength in the abdominal and back muscles.

SITUPS (ABDOMINAL STRENGTH): SKILL LEVEL 3

Performance Objective

The child with acquisition of Skill Level 2 or a level of performance appropriate for the child's level of functioning can maintain that level over six weeks.

Given activities that require the skill, the child can

1. play two or more games listed below at home or school, and
2. play with equipment selected by teacher and parent(s).

Skills to Review

1. Level 1 situp. Take a starting position (lying on back, knees bent 90 degrees, feet flat on mat, arms at sides, feet supported), then
2. curl up by tucking chin and lifting shoulders (upper back) off the mat and
3. return to starting position in controlled movement by uncurling and lowering head to mat.
4. Level 2 situp. Curl up by tucking chin and lifting trunk, complete curl by touching knees with hands and
5. return in controlled manner by uncurling trunk and lowering head to mat, hands on thighs, and then
6. repeat ten times (or meet standards appropriate for the child).

Action Words

Actions: Bend, control, curl, lie, lift, raise, return, sit, tuck, uncurl

Objects: Arm, back, chin, drum, foot, floor, hand, head, knee, mat, shoulder, toy

Concepts: Down, flat, look, ready, show me, up, upper

Games

- Beat the Stars
- Did You Ever See a Lassie/Laddie?
- Follow the Leader
- Obstacle Course
- Simon Says
- Trunk Lifts

TEACHING ACTIVITIES FOR MAINTENANCE

In Teaching

1. Provide the child with teaching cues (verbal and nonverbal, such as demonstration, modeling, imitating) for situps that involve the skill components the child has achieved in compatible teaching and play activities. Bring to the child's attention the skill components he or she has already achieved. Provide positive reinforcement and feedback for the child.
2. Use games that require situps and that involve imitating, modeling, and demonstrating.
3. Observe and assess each child's maintenance at the end of two weeks. Repeat at the end of four weeks (if maintained) and six weeks after initial date of attainment.

▲ Box in the skill level to be maintained on the child's Class Record of Progress. Note the date the child attained target level of performance (defined by teacher alone or co-planned with parents).

▲ Two weeks after attainment, observe the child. Is the level maintained? If child does not demonstrate the skill components at the desired level of performance, indicate the skill components that need reteaching or reinforcing in the comments sheet on the Class Record of Progress. Reschedule teaching time, and co-plan with parents the home activities necessary to reinforce child's achievement of the skill components and maintenance of attainment.

▲ Continue to observe the child, and reteach and reinforce until the child maintains that level of performance for six weeks.

▲ Plan teaching activities incorporating these components so that the child can continually use and reinforce them and can acquire new ones over the year.

▲ When the child can understand it, make a checklist poster illustrating the child's achievements. Bring the child's attention to these skill components in various compatible play and game activities throughout the year. Have the child help others—a partner or a small group.

In Co-Planning with Parent(s)

1. Encourage the parent(s) to reinforce the child's achievement of the skill components in everyday play and living activities in the home.

▲ Provide key action words for the parent(s) to emphasize.

▲ Give the parent(s) a list of play and games to use in playing with the child, thus reinforcing the skill components the child has achieved and needs support to maintain.

▲ Give the parent(s) a list of abdominal strength activities that can be done at home with the child, such as

　　a. Playing Beat the Stars with your best friend and winning.

　　b. Running the park obstacle course and doing situps at the correct stations.

　　c. Performing ten situps as a warm-up exercise before you run or walk around the block or hang or climb on play equipment.

　　d. Performing situps without someone holding your feet.

　　e. Variation: Situps on various surfaces (floor, mat, grass, mattress).

2. Set up a time every two weeks to interact with the parent(s) and exchange feedback on the child's progress.

WALK-RUN FOR ENDURANCE: SKILL LEVEL 1

Performance Objective

The child with ability to walk can perform an endurance walk-run three consecutive times, demonstrating the following skill components:

Within a clear space of 100 feet, the child can

1. walk-run continuously in any manner at moderate to fast pace for one minute and then

2. walk-run continuously in any manner for three minutes.

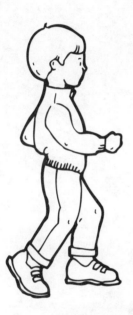 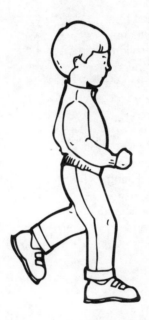 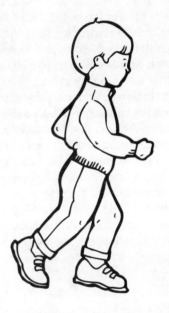

Action Words

Actions: Go, run, step, stop, walk

Objects: Arm, bases, cones, drum, foot, line, tape, toy

Concepts: Fast, forward, look, ready, show me, slow

Games

- Around the World
- Base Running
- Endurance Course
- Figure 8 Run
- Follow the Leader
- Obstacle Course
- Walk-Run Relay

TEACHING ACTIVITIES

If a child requires assistance to respond,

1. give verbal cues and physical assistance.
Assist by standing behind or in front of the child, grasping the child's arm, and walking the course together. Give the child specific verbal instructions throughout (in sign language, bliss symbols, action cues), such as "Keep walking," "Walk the course," "Ready, set, go."

2. give verbal cues with demonstration.
Use a model or have the child watch you walk the course with the other children. Then have the child perform the action. Use specific verbal instructions (as in 1 above with the modeling).

If a child can respond without assistance,

3. give a verbal challenge in the form of a problem: "Who can . . . ?" "Show me how you can . . ."

a. Walk the square course and follow the taped lines.

b. Walk the course when I blow the whistle; stop when I blow the whistle again.

c. Walk the course and get the reward (drink, food, token) at the end of the walk.

d. Variation: Walk to beat of drum.

4. introduce self-initiated learning activities.
Set up the equipment and space for walk-running. Provide time at the beginning of the lesson and free time for independent learning after the child understands the skills to be used. You may ask the child to create a game activity to play alone or with others (partner or small group) on or around the equipment.

5. Variations: Set up an obstacle course that includes colored tape. Play a game, such as Base Running, Around the World, or Endurance Course, that incorporates walk-run activities for endurance. Run in place. Run to music. Health fitness activities such as walking, running, skipping, galloping, biking, and swimming are also important movements in developing heart-lung endurance. Many rhythmic and dance activities that are continuous in nature and involve moving the body are also important.

WALK-RUN FOR ENDURANCE: SKILL LEVEL 2

Performance Objective

The child with acquisition of Skill Level 1 endurance and the ability to walk-run can walk-run for endurance three consecutive times, demonstrating the following skill components:

Within a clear space of 100 feet, the child can

3. walk-run for two minutes (with two or more periods of nonsupport every ten steps) and then

4. walk-run for four minutes (with two or more periods of nonsupport every ten steps).

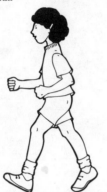 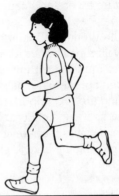

Skills to Review

1. Walk-run continuously in any manner at moderate to fast pace for one minute and then

2. Walk-run continuously in any manner at moderate to fast pace for three minutes.

Action Words

Actions: Go, run, step, stop, walk

Objects: Arm, bases, cones, drum, foot, line, tape, toy

Concepts: Fast, forward, look, ready, show me, slow

Games

- Around the World
- Base Running
- Endurance Course
- Figure 8 Run
- Follow the Leader
- Obstacle Course
- Walk-Run Relay

TEACHING ACTIVITIES

If a child requires assistance to respond,

1. give verbal cues and physical assistance.
Assist by standing behind or in front of the child, grasping the child's arm, and walking the course together. Give the child specific verbal instructions throughout (in sign language, bliss symbols, action cues), such as "Keep walking," "Walk the course," "Ready, set, go."

2. give verbal cues with demonstration.
Use a model or have the child watch you walk the course with the other children. Then have the child perform the action. Use specific verbal instructions (as in 1 above with the modeling).

If a child can respond without assistance,

3. give a verbal challenge in the form of a problem: "Who can . . . ?" "Show me how you can . . ."

a. Walk the square course and follow the taped lines.

b. Walk the course when I blow the whistle; stop when I blow the whistle again.

c. Walk the course and get the reward (drink, food, token) at the end of the walk.

d. Variation: Walk to beat of drum.

4. introduce self-initiated learning activities.
Set up the equipment and space for walk-running.
Provide time at the beginning of the lesson and
free time for independent learning after the child
understands the skills to be used. You may ask the
child to create a game activity to play alone or with
others (partner or small group) on or around the
equipment.

5. Variations: Set up an obstacle course that
includes colored tape. Play a game, such as Base
Running, Around the World, or Endurance Course,
that incorporates walk-run activities for endurance.
Run in place. Run to music. Health fitness activities
such as walking, running, skipping, galloping,
biking, and swimming are also important movements in developing heart-lung endurance. Many
rhythmic and dance activities that are continuous in
nature and involve moving the body are also
important.

WALK-RUN FOR ENDURANCE: SKILL LEVEL 3

Performance Objective

The child with acquisition of Skill Level 2 or a level of performance appropriate for the child's level of functioning can maintain that level over six weeks.

Given activities that require the skill, the child can

1. play two or more games listed below at home or school, and
2. play with equipment selected by teacher and parent(s).

Skills to Review

1. Level 1 walk-run. Walk-run continuously in any manner at moderate to fast pace for one minute and then
2. walk-run continuously in any manner at moderate to fast pace for three minutes.
3. Level 2 walk-run. Walk-run for two minutes (with two or more periods of nonsupport every ten steps) and then
4. walk-run for four minutes (with two or more periods of nonsupport every ten steps).

Action Words

Actions: Go, run, step, stop, walk

Objects: Arm, bases, cones, drum, foot, line, tape, toy

Concepts: Fast, forward, look, ready, show me, slow

Games

- Around the World
- Base Running
- Endurance Course
- Figure 8 Run
- Follow the Leader
- Obstacle Course
- Walk-Run Relay

TEACHING ACTIVITIES FOR MAINTENANCE

In Teaching

1. Provide the child with teaching cues (verbal and nonverbal, such as demonstration, modeling, imitating) for walk-run that involve the skill components the child has achieved in compatible teaching and play activities. Bring to the child's attention the skill components he or she has already achieved. Provide positive reinforcement and feedback for the child.

2. Use games that require walk-running and that involve imitating, modeling, and demonstrating.

3. Observe and assess each child's maintenance at the end of two weeks. Repeat at the end of four weeks (if maintained) and six weeks after initial date of attainment.

▲ Box in the skill level to be maintained on the child's Class Record of Progress. Note the date the child attained target level of performance (defined by teacher alone or co-planned with parents).

▲ Two weeks after attainment, observe the child. Is the level maintained? If child does not demonstrate the skill components at the desired level of performance, indicate the skill components that need reteaching or reinforcing in the comments sheet on the Class Record of Progress. Reschedule teaching time, and co-plan with parents the home activities necessary to reinforce child's achievement of the skill components and maintenance of attainment.

▲ Continue to observe the child, and reteach and reinforce until the child maintains that level of performance for six weeks.

▲ Plan teaching activities incorporating these components so that the child can continually use and reinforce them and can acquire new ones over the year.

▲ When the child can understand it, make a checklist poster illustrating the child's achievements. Bring the child's attention to these skill components in various compatible play and game activities throughout the year. Have the child help others—a partner or a small group.

In Co-Planning with Parent(s)

1. Encourage the parent(s) to reinforce the child's achievement of the skill components in everyday play and living activities in the home.

▲ Provide key action words for the parent(s) to emphasize.

▲ Give the parent(s) a list of play and games to use in playing with the child, thus reinforcing the skill components the child has achieved and needs support to maintain.

▲ Give the parent(s) a list of endurance activities that can be done at home with the child, such as

   a. Playing Base Running with friends and seeing how many times you can run the bases.

   b. Timing a walk-run on an endurance course at the local park.

   c. Walk-running on the beach.

   d. Walk-running on the nature hike at local park.

   e. Walk-running to the top of a large hill.

   f. Variations: Walk-running on various terrains (grass, cement, sand, dirt)—which can you move fastest on?

2. Set up a time every two weeks to interact with the parent(s) and exchange feedback on the child's progress.

TRUNK AND LEG FLEXIBILITY: SKILL LEVEL 1

Performance Objective

The child with ability to sit and bend forward can sit-reach three consecutive times, demonstrating the following skill components:

With a sit-and-reach bench (with measuring stick on top of bench), the child can

1. take starting position (sitting on the floor, legs straight, feet flat against sit-and-reach bench or wall, hands on front of thighs, and

2. bend forward, reach with hands toward bench or wall with legs straight, hold for three seconds, and return to starting position.

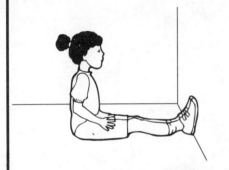 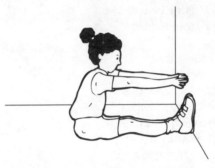 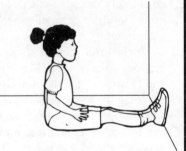

Action Words

Actions: Bend, hold, reach, return, sit, start

Objects: Arm, bench, box, footprints, hand, leg, stick, toy, yardstick

Concepts: Flat, forward, front, look, ready, show me, slowly, straight

Games

- Follow the Leader
- Giants and Dwarfs
- Obstacle Course
- Shuttle Run Relay
- Simon Says
- Trunk and Leg Relay

TEACHING ACTIVITIES

If a child requires assistance to respond,

1. give verbal cues and physical assistance.
Have the child sit on the floor with feet flat against the bench (or box), legs straight. With one hand, hold the child's knees; with other hand, hold both of the child's hands and slowly pull them toward the bench. Hold the toes for at least five seconds. Give the child specific verbal instructions throughout (in sign language, bliss symbols, action cues), such as "Sit down," "Put your feet against the bench (box), slowly reach for the bench," "Ready, go."

2. give verbal cues with demonstration.
Use a model or have the child watch you sit and reach. Emphasize starting with feet flat against bench, legs straight, then bending forward and reaching toward bench. Hold for five seconds; return to start. Then have the child perform the action. Use specific verbal instructions (as in 1 above with the modeling).

If a child can respond without assistance,

3. **give a verbal challenge in the form of a problem: "Who can . . . ?" "Show me how you can . . ."**

   a. Sit and reach the picture on the bench.

   b. Sit and reach to touch your feet. How long can you hold them?

   c. Sit and reach to grab the toy on the box.

   d. Variations: Sit and reach to beat of drum. Use footprints on the bench to show foot position.

4. **introduce self-initiated learning activities.** Set up the equipment and space for trunk-leg flexibility. Provide time at the beginning of the lesson and free time for independent learning after the child understands the skills to be used. You may ask the child to create a game activity to play alone or with others (partner or small group) on or around the equipment.

5. **Variations:** Set up an obstacle course that includes colored tape. Play a game, such as Giants and Dwarfs or Shuttle Run Relay, that incorporates trunk-leg flexibility activities. Health fitness activities such as bending, turning, twisting, hanging, stretching, and climbing are also important movements in developing and maintaining flexibility. Rhythmic and body management activities that involve turning, twisting, bending, and stretching also help to develop and maintain flexibility.

Performance Objective

The child with acquisition of Skill Level 1 can sit-reach three consecutive times, demonstrating the following skill components:

With a bench or wall space, the child can

3. bend forward, reach with hands toward sit-and-reach bench or wall, hold five seconds, and return to starting position, and then

4. bend forward and touch wall or reach a measurement on sit-and-reach bench established as appropriate for the child.

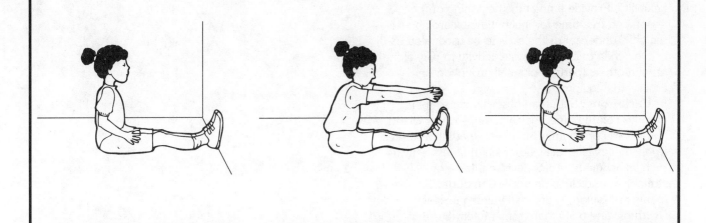

Skills to Review

1. Take starting position (sitting on floor, legs straight, feet against sit-and-reach bench or wall), hands on front of thighs, and

2. bend forward, reach with hands toward bench or wall with legs straight, hold for three seconds, and return to starting position.

Action Words

Actions: Bend, hold, reach, return, sit, start

Objects: Arm, bench, box, footprints, hand, leg, stick, toy, yardstick

Concepts: Flat, forward, front, look, ready, show me, slowly, straight

Games

- Follow the Leader
- Giants and Dwarfs
- Obstacle Course
- Shuttle Run Relay
- Simon Says
- Trunk and Leg Relay

TEACHING ACTIVITIES

If a child requires assistance to respond,

1. give verbal cues and physical assistance.
Have the child sit on the floor with feet flat against the bench (or box), legs straight. With one hand, hold the child's knees; with other hand, hold both of the child's hands and slowly pull them toward the bench. Have the child reach as far as possible, and measure distance the hands reach beyond toes. Give the child specific verbal instructions throughout (in sign language, bliss symbols, action cues), such as "Ready," "Reach," "Hold your hands there."

2. give verbal cues with demonstration.
Use a model or have the child watch you demonstrate the correct action of the sit and reach. Emphasize beginning on the cue "Reach." Hold as far as you can until your reach is measured. Then have the child perform the action. Use specific verbal instructions (as in 1 above with the modeling).

If a child can respond without assistance,

3. **give a verbal challenge in the form of a problem: "Who can . . . ?" "Show me how you can . . ."**

   a. How far can you reach past your toes?

   b. Reach farther than you did before.

   c. Reach for the toy way beyond your toes on the bench.

   d. Variations: Sit and reach to beat of drum. Hold it when the drum stops; return to sitting when drum starts again.

4. **introduce self-initiated learning activities.** Set up the equipment and space for trunk-leg flexibility. Provide time at the beginning of the lesson and free time for independent learning after the child understands the skills to be used. You may ask the child to create a game activity to play alone or with others (partner or small group) on or around the equipment.

5. **Variations:** Set up an obstacle course that includes colored tape. Play a game, such as Giants and Dwarfs or Shuttle Run Relay, that incorporates trunk-leg flexibility activities. Health fitness activities such as bending, turning, twisting, hanging, stretching, and climbing are also important movements in developing and maintaining flexibility. Rhythmic and body management activities that involve turning, twisting, bending, and stretching also help to develop and maintain flexibility.

Performance Objective

The child with acquisition of Skill Level 2 or a level of performance appropriate for the child's level of functioning can maintain that level over six weeks.

Given activities that require the skill, the child can

1. play two or more games listed below at home or school, and
2. play with equipment selected by teacher and parent(s).

Skills to Review

1. Level 1 flexibility. Take starting position (sitting on floor, legs straight, feet against sit-and-reach bench or wall), hands on front of thighs, and
2. bend forward, reach with hands toward bench or wall with legs straight, hold for three seconds, and return to starting position.
3. Level 2 flexibility. Bend forward, reach with hands toward sit-and-reach bench or wall, hold five seconds, and return to starting position, and then
4. bend forward and touch wall or reach measurement on sit-and-reach bench established as appropriate for child.

Action Words

Actions: Bend, hold, reach, return, sit, start

Objects: Arm, bench, box, footprints, hand, leg, stick, toy, yardstick

Concepts: Flat, forward, front, look, ready, show me, slowly, straight

Games

- Follow the Leader
- Giants and Dwarfs
- Obstacle Course
- Shuttle Run Relay
- Simon Says
- Trunk and Leg Relay

TEACHING ACTIVITIES FOR MAINTENANCE

In Teaching

1. Provide the child with teaching cues (verbal and nonverbal, such as demonstration, modeling, imitating) for trunk and leg flexibility that involve the skill components the child has achieved in compatible teaching and play activities. Bring to the child's attention the skill components he or she has already achieved. Provide positive reinforcement and feedback for the child.
2. Use games that require trunk and leg flexibility and that involve imitating, modeling, and demonstrating.
3. Observe and assess each child's maintenance at the end of two weeks. Repeat at the end of four weeks (if maintained) and six weeks after initial date of attainment.

▲ Box in the skill level to be maintained on the child's Class Record of Progress. Note the date the child attained target level of performance (defined by teacher alone or co-planned with parents).

▲ Two weeks after attainment, observe the child. Is the level maintained? If child does not demonstrate the skill components at the desired level of performance, indicate the skill components that need reteaching or reinforcing in the comments sheet on the Class Record of Progress. Reschedule teaching time, and co-plan with parents the home activities necessary to reinforce child's achievement of the skill components and maintenance of attainment.

▲ Continue to observe the child, and reteach and reinforce until the child maintains that level of performance for six weeks.

▲ Plan teaching activities incorporating these components so that the child can continually use and reinforce them and can acquire new ones over the year.

▲ When the child can understand it, make a checklist poster illustrating the child's achievements. Bring the child's attention to these skill components in various compatible play and game activities throughout the year. Have the child help others—a partner or a small group.

In Co-Planning with Parent(s)

1. Encourage the parent(s) to reinforce the child's achievement of the skill components in everyday play and living activities in the home.

▲ Provide key action words for the parent(s) to emphasize.

▲ Give the parent(s) a list of play and games to use in playing with the child, thus reinforcing the skill components the child has achieved and needs support to maintain.

▲ Give the parent(s) a list of bending and stretching activities that can be done at home with the child, such as

a. Bending and stretching exercises in bed.

b. Performing sit-reach-hold as warm-up when getting up or going to bed.

c. Performing sit-reach-hold with feet placed against wall.

d. Sitting on the floor, bending forward, and putting on shoes.

2. Set up a time every two weeks to interact with the parent(s) and exchange feedback on the child's progress.

LIFT AND CARRY OBJECTS: SKILL LEVEL 1

Performance Objective

The child with ability to bend knees, maintain balance, and grasp an object can lift an object (1–2 lbs. or less) from the floor with two hands three consecutive times, demonstrating the following skill components:

Within a clear space of 10 feet, the child can

1. position body close to object to be lifted, with weight on both feet evenly distributed, then
2. bend knees and lower body, keeping back straight, and grasp object with both hands and
3. lift object by straightening legs, keeping back straight.

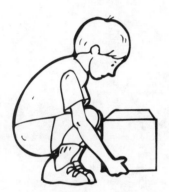 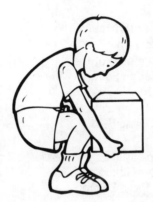 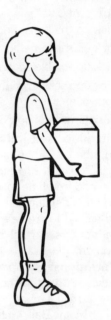

Action Words

Actions: Bend, carry, grasp, hold, lean, lift, move, pick up, stand, step

Objects: Back, block, box, feet, hand, knee, leg, toy

Concepts: Backward, both, close, forward, look, ready, show me, side, straight, up

Games

- Follow the Leader
- Lift a Box
- Lift and Pass
- Line Carry
- Magic Ball
- Medicine Ball
- Moving Game
- Obstacle Course
- Scatter Play

TEACHING ACTIVITIES

If a child requires assistance to respond,

1. give verbal cues and physical assistance.
Grasp child's shoulders or waist and move the child's body so that it is close to the object to be lifted. Position the child so that weight is *evenly* distributed on both feet by pushing him or her first on front foot and then on back foot. Bend the child's knees so that body is lowered, and assist child in lifting the object so that body weight is over knees. Give the child specific verbal instructions throughout (in sign language, bliss symbols, action cues), such as "Stand close to the box," "Bend your knees," "Lift the box."

2. give verbal cues with demonstration.
Use a model or have the child watch you lift object by positioning yourself close to the object, keeping weight evenly distributed. Flex knees to lower body center of gravity toward object. Use thighs as primary movers to raise object. Then have the child perform the action. Use specific verbal instructions (as in 1 above with the modeling).

If a child can respond without assistance,

3. give a verbal challenge in the form of a problem: "Who can . . . ?" "Show me how you can . . ."

a. Pick up the large block and move it here.

b. Pick up the large box and bring it to me.

c. Pick up the blocks one at a time and build a tower.

d. Pick up rocks from the ground and carry them in your bag.

e. Variation: Pick up objects to beat of drum.

4. introduce self-initiated learning activities.
Set up the equipment and space for lifting and carrying objects. Provide time at the beginning of the lesson and free time for independent learning after the child understands the skills to be used. You may ask the child to create a game activity to play alone or with others (partner or small group), using the equipment.

5. Variations: Set up an obstacle course that includes colored tape and mats to perform lifting and carrying. Play a game, such as Lift and Pass, Scatter Play, or Magic Ball. Getting out, cleaning, and putting equipment away provide everyday activities for teaching and practicing this skill.

Performance Objective

The child with acquisition of Skill Level 1 can hold and carry an object (1–5 lbs.) three consecutive times, demonstrating the following skill components:

Within a clear space of 10 feet, the child can

4. bend elbows slightly to hold object as close to body as possible in lifting and carrying and

5. keep head, shoulders, and back straight in standing posture alignment and then

6. carry object with both hands close to body for 10 feet, lower object to floor in correct manner (described in skill components 1 and 2).

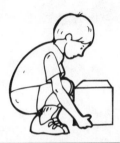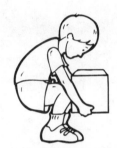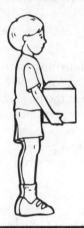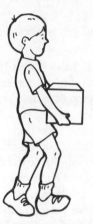

Skills to Review

1. Position body close to object to be lifted, with weight on both feet evenly distributed, then

2. bend knees and lower body, keeping back straight, and grasp object with both hands and

3. lift object by straightening legs, keeping back straight.

Action Words

Actions: Bend, carry, grasp, hold, lean, lift, move, pick up, stand, step

Objects: Back, block, box, feet, hand, knee, leg, toy

Concepts: Backward, both, close, forward, look, ready, show me, side, straight, up

Games

- Follow the Leader
- Lift a Box
- Lift and Pass
- Lifting Relay
- Line Carry
- Magic Ball
- Medicine Ball
- Moving Game
- Obstacle Course
- Scatter Play

TEACHING ACTIVITIES

If a child requires assistance to respond,

1. give verbal cues and physical assistance.
Face the child in standing position. Place object in front of child. Grasp child's waist and hands, and pull them down in front of child to grasp box. Have the child begin walking, and manipulate the child's hips, head, and shoulders in same manner as his or her walk. Grasp child's upper arms and elbows. Pull on the arms to bend them. As the child walks, keep your hand on the elbows to keep box near the center of gravity. Give the child specific verbal instructions throughout (in sign language, bliss symbols, action cues), such as "Hold the box with two hands," "Walk with it," "Stand straight," "Bend your elbows," "Keep the box close to you."

2. give verbal cues with demonstration.
Use a model or have the child watch you demonstrate how to lift and carry large objects with two hands by keeping head, shoulders, and hips aligned as in standing. With elbows slightly bent, hold object close to body's center of gravity. Walk 20 feet with the 5–10 lb. weight. Then have the child perform the action. Use specific verbal instructions (as in 1 above with the modeling).

If a child can respond without assistance,

3. **give a verbal challenge in the form of a problem: "Who can . . . ?" "Show me how you can . . ."**

   a. Pick up the books and put them away on the shelf.

   b. Pick up the blocks and put them in the corner.

   c. Pick up the containers of water and carry them to the sink without dropping them.

   d. Pick up the toys in the bathtub and bring them to me.

   e. Variation: Pick up and carry objects to beat of drum.

4. **introduce self-initiated learning activities.** Set up the equipment and space for lifting and carrying objects. Provide time at the beginning of the lesson and free time for independent learning after the child understands the skills to be used. You may ask the child to create a game activity to play alone or with others (partner or small group), using the equipment.

5. **Variations:** Set up an obstacle course that includes colored tape and mats to perform lifting and carrying. Play a game, such as Lift and Pass, Scatter Play, or Magic Ball. Getting out, cleaning, and putting equipment away provide everyday activities for teaching and practicing this skill.

Performance Objective

The child with acquisition of Skill Level 2 or a level of performance appropriate for the child's level of functioning can maintain that level over six weeks.

Given activities that require the skill, the child can

1. play two or more games listed below at home or school, and
2. play with equipment selected by teacher and parent(s).

Skills to Review

1. Level 1 lift and carry. Position body close to object to be lifted, with weight on both feet evenly distributed, then
2. bend knees and lower body, keeping back straight, and grasp object with both hands and
3. lift object by straightening legs, keeping back straight.
4. Level 2 lift and carry. Bend elbows slightly to hold object as close to body as possible in lifting and carrying and
5. keep head, shoulders, and back straight in standing posture alignment and then
6. carry object with both hands close to body for 10 feet, lower object to floor in correct manner (described in skill components 1 and 2).

Action Words

Actions: Bend, carry, grasp, hold, lean, lift, move, pick up, stand, step

Objects: Back, block, box, feet, hand, knee, leg, toy

Concepts: Backward, both, close, forward, look, ready, show me, side, straight, up

Games

- Follow the Leader
- Lift a Box
- Lift and Pass
- Lifting Relay
- Line Carry
- Magic Ball
- Medicine Ball
- Moving Game
- Obstacle Course
- Scatter Play

TEACHING ACTIVITIES FOR MAINTENANCE

In Teaching

1. Provide the child with teaching cues (verbal and nonverbal, such as demonstration, modeling, imitating) for lifting and carrying objects that involve the skill components the child has achieved in compatible teaching and play activities. Bring to the child's attention the skill components he or she has already achieved. Provide positive reinforcement and feedback for the child.

2. Use games that require lifting and carrying objects and that involve imitating, modeling, and demonstrating.

3. Observe and assess each child's maintenance at the end of two weeks. Repeat at the end of four weeks (if maintained) and six weeks after initial date of attainment.

▲ Box in the skill level to be maintained on the child's Class Record of Progress. Note the date the child attained target level of performance (defined by teacher alone or co-planned with parents).

▲ Two weeks after attainment, observe the child. Is the level maintained? If child does not demonstrate the skill components at the desired level of performance, indicate the skill components that need reteaching or reinforcing in the comments sheet on the Class Record of Progress. Reschedule teaching time, and co-plan with parents the home activities necessary to reinforce child's achievement of the skill components and maintenance of attainment.

▲ Continue to observe the child, and reteach and reinforce until the child maintains that level of performance for six weeks.

▲ Plan teaching activities incorporating these components so that the child can continually use and reinforce them and can acquire new ones over the year.

▲ When the child can understand it, make a checklist poster illustrating the child's achievements. Bring the child's attention to these skill components in various compatible play and game activities throughout the year. Have the child help others—a partner or a small group.

In Co-Planning with Parent(s)

1. Encourage the parent(s) to reinforce the child's achievement of the skill components in everyday play and living activities in the home.

▲ Provide key action words for the parent(s) to emphasize.

▲ Give the parent(s) a list of play and games to use in playing with the child, thus reinforcing the skill components the child has achieved and needs support to maintain.

▲ Give the parent(s) a list of lifting and carrying activities that can be done at home with the child, such as
   a. Picking up the loaf of bread and putting it in the grocery cart.
   b. Picking up the picture from the floor and giving it to me.
   c. Reaching down into the wading pool and picking up the block.
   d. Picking up the chalk and taking it to the wall.
   e. Picking up the books and carrying them over to the shelf.
   f. Picking up your lunch box and carrying it to school.
   g. Picking up the dirty plastic dishes from the table and carrying them to the sink.
   h. Picking up the puppy and carrying it to its bed.
   i. Picking up the trash and carrying it outside.
   j. Playing Scatter Play and finding five objects.
   k. Playing Lift and Pass and passing objects of various sizes.

2. Set up a time every two weeks to interact with the parent(s) and exchange feedback on the child's progress.

REST AND RELAXATION: SKILL LEVEL 1

Performance Objective

The child with ability to relax (on back, sitting) can recognize muscular tension in body parts three consecutive times, demonstrating the following skill components:

On an 8-foot mat in quiet-time space, the child can

1. lie on back, arms at sides, legs apart, eyes closed, head turned to left or right (or sit in a chair or a position appropriate for the child) and

2. recognize muscular tension in four or more body parts (head turning from side to side, eyes squeezed closed, lips tight, jaw clenched, face frowning, breathing fast or holding breath, arms turned in or moving, fist clenched or fingers moving, legs turned in or moving, foot rigid or moving, toes curled or rigid).

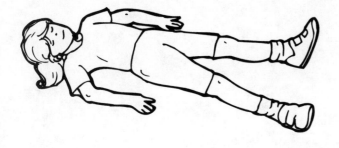

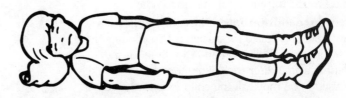

Action Words

Actions: Bend, breathing, fist, hold, squeeze tight

Objects: Arm, eyes, face, fingers, foot, hand, head, leg, mat, toes

Concepts: Down, feel, forward, hard, let go, look, ready, relax, show me, slowly, tense, up

Games

- Do What I Do
- Follow the Leader
- I Am a Balloon
- Jello Jiggle
- Let's Relax
- Obstacle Course
- Raggedy Ann and Andy
- Simon Says
- Stretch and Relax
- ZZZZ

TEACHING ACTIVITIES

If a child requires assistance to respond,

1. give verbal cues and physical assistance.
Move the child's head so that there is alternating tensing and relaxing, or letting go.

a. Move one part at a time: arm at shoulder, at elbow, at hand. Then move the leg at hip, at knee, at foot.

b. Have the child tense different parts of the body: turn head from side to side and hold, let go; turn arms in and out; turn legs in and out; push foot down and up; clench hand, making a fist and letting go.

c. Have child sit in chair or on ground. Let head drop slowly back, and then lift head slowly forward. Return to starting position. Repeat with shoulders. Shrug shoulders. Let drop. Return to starting position.

Give the child specific verbal instructions throughout (in sign language, bliss symbols, action cues). Create images of loose and floppy, tight and tense. Suggest different animals, such as cat asleep or seeing a dog. Use dolls, such as a Raggedy Ann Doll.

2. give verbal cues with demonstration.
Use a model or have the child watch you tense different body parts. Frown. Close eyes tightly. Clench fist. Hold breathing. Breathe fast. Then demonstrate relaxing a body part. Then have the child perform the actions. Use specific verbal instructions (as in 1 above with the modeling).

If a child can respond without assistance,

3. give a verbal challenge in the form of a problem: "Who can . . . ?" "Show me how you can . . ."

a. Tense your arms and legs. Then relax, or let go.

b. Shrug your shoulders. Then relax, or let go.

c. Bend forward, let your arms be floppy. Relax.

d. Variations: Tense and relax body parts to music— harsh music to tense, soft music to relax.

4. introduce self-initiated learning activities.
Set up mats and space for relaxing. Provide time at the beginning of the lesson and free time for independent learning after the child understands the skills to be used. You may ask the child to create a game activity to play alone or with others (partner or small group) on the carpet squares or mats.

5. Variations: Set up mats for a specified time of relaxation. Play a game, such as Let's Relax, Jello Jiggle, or ZZZZ, that incorporates relaxation and recognition of muscle tension in different body parts.

REST AND RELAXATION: SKILL LEVEL 2

Performance Objective

The child with acquisition of Skill Level 1 (recognizes muscular tension) can release muscle tension in different body parts three consecutive times, demonstrating the following skill components:

On an 8-foot mat in quiet-time space, the child can

3. relax four or more body parts for one minute, beginning with the head, face, eyes, and jaw, then

4. relax other body parts until total body is relaxed (breathing, arms, hands, legs, feet, and toes), and then

5. relax total body for one minute or more.

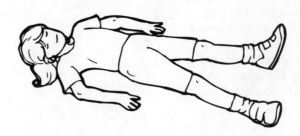

Skills to Review

1. Lie on back, arms at sides, legs apart, *eyes closed*, head turned to left or right (or sit in chair or position appropriate for child) and

2. recognize muscular tension in four or more body parts (head turning from side to side, eyes squeezed closed, lips tight, jaw clenched, breathing fast or holding breath, arms turned in or moving, fist clenched or fingers moving, legs turned in or moving, foot rigid or moving, toes curled or rigid).

Action Words

Actions: Bend, breathing, fist, hold, squeeze tight

Objects: Arm, eyes, face, fingers, foot, hand, head, leg, mat, toes

Concepts: Down, feel, forward, hard, let go, look, ready, relax, show me, slowly, tense up

Games

- Do What I Do
- Follow the Leader
- I Am a Balloon
- Jello Jiggle
- Let's Relax
- Obstacle Course
- Raggedy Ann and Andy
- Simon Says
- Stretch and Relax
- ZZZZ

TEACHING ACTIVITIES

If a child requires assistance to respond,

1. give verbal cues and physical assistance.
Have child lie on back with eyes closed. Place child's arms by side (but not touching), and move the child's legs apart. Manipulate one body part at a time. Lift child's head from floor, and have child hold this position, then return head to floor. When child can relax head, clench his or her fists. Then have child hold hands unclenched. Gradually add all body parts until child can relax total body. Touch body part that child still needs to relax. Relax for two minutes. Play soft music to set atmosphere for relaxing.

2. give verbal cues with demonstration.
Use a model or have the child watch you relax body parts one at a time (head to toe) until total body is relaxed. Do this for two minutes. Then have the child perform the action. Use specific verbal instructions (as in 1 above with the modeling).

If a child can respond without assistance,

3. give a verbal challenge in the form of a problem: "Who can . . . ?" "Show me how you can . . ."

a. Relax your whole body. Pretend your body is floating on a cloud.

b. Relax your whole body. Pretend your body is sitting in the sand.

c. Tense your whole body (make your muscles hard), beginning with your head down to toes. Then let your body go limp like a rag doll.

d. Variation: Tense and relax different body parts to music.

4. introduce self-initiated learning activities. Set up mats and space for relaxation. Provide time at the beginning of the lesson and free time for independent learning after the child understands the skills to be used. You may ask the child to create a game activity to play alone or with others (partner or small group) on carpet squares or mats.

5. Variations: Set up mats for specified time of relaxation. Play a game, such as Let's Relax, Jello Jiggle, or ZZZZ, that incorporates relaxation and recognition of muscle tension in different body parts.

REST AND RELAXATION: SKILL LEVEL 3

Performance Objective

The child with acquisition of Skill Level 2 or a level of performance appropriate for the child's level of functioning can maintain that level over six weeks.

Given activities that require the skill, the child can

1. play two or more games listed below at home or school, and
2. play with equipment selected by teacher and parent(s).

Skills to Review

1. Level 1 relaxation. Lie on back, arms at sides, legs apart, eyes closed, head turned to left or right (or sit in chair or position appropriate for child) and
2. recognize muscular tension in four or more body parts (head turning from side to side, eyes squeezed closed, lips tight, jaw clenched, breathing fast or holding breath, arms turned in or moving, fist clenched or fingers moving, legs turned in or moving, foot rigid or moving, toes curled or rigid).
3. Level 2 relaxation. Relax four or more body parts for one minute, beginning with head, face, eyes, and jaw, then
4. relax other body parts until total body is relaxed (breathing, arms, hands, legs, feet, and toes), and then
5. relax total body for one minute or more.

Action Words

Actions: Bend, breathing, fist, hold, squeeze tight

Objects: Arm, eyes, face, fingers, foot, hand, head, leg, mat, toes

Concepts: Down, feel, forward, hard, let go, look, ready, relax, show me, slowly, tense, up

Games

- Do What I Do
- Follow the Leader
- I Am a Balloon
- Jello Jiggle
- Let's Relax
- Obstacle Course
- Raggedy Ann and Andy
- Simon Says
- Stretch and Relax
- ZZZZ

TEACHING ACTIVITIES FOR MAINTENANCE

In Teaching

1. Provide the child with teaching cues (verbal and nonverbal, such as demonstration, modeling, imitating) for relaxation that involve the skill components the child has achieved in compatible teaching and play activities. Bring to the child's attention the skill components he or she has already achieved. Provide positive reinforcement and feedback for the child.

2. Use games that require relaxing and that involve imitating, modeling, and demonstrating.

3. Observe and assess each child's maintenance at the end of two weeks. Repeat at the end of four weeks (if maintained) and six weeks after initial date of attainment.

▲ Box in the skill level to be maintained on the child's Class Record of Progress. Note the date the child attained target level of performance (defined by teacher alone or co-planned with parents).

▲ Two weeks after attainment, observe the child. Is the level maintained? If child does not demonstrate the skill components at the desired level of performance, indicate the skill components that need reteaching or reinforcing in the comments sheet on the Class Record of Progress. Reschedule teaching time, and co-plan with parents the home activities necessary to reinforce child's achievement of the skill components and maintenance of attainment.

▲ Continue to observe the child, and reteach and reinforce until the child maintains that level of performance for six weeks.

▲ Plan teaching activities incorporating these components so that the child can continually use and reinforce them and can acquire new ones over the year.

▲ When the child can understand it, make a check-list poster illustrating the child's achievements. Bring the child's attention to these skill components in various compatible play and game activities throughout the year. Have the child help others—a partner or a small group.

In Co-Planning with Parent(s)

1. Encourage the parent(s) to reinforce the child's achievement of the skill components in everyday play and living activities in the home.

▲ Provide key action words for the parent(s) to emphasize.

▲ Give the parent(s) a list of play and games to use in playing with the child, thus reinforcing the skill components the child has achieved and needs support to maintain.

▲ Give the parent(s) a list of relaxation activities that can be done at home with the child, such as
   a. Relaxing and reading a book on the couch.
   b. Resting on a hammock in the sun while listening to the radio.
   c. Painting a picture to music.
   d. Playing Let's Relax with group of friends.
   e. Playing ZZZZ with your best friend.

2. Set up a time every two weeks to interact with the parent(s) and exchange feedback on the child's progress.

Checklists:
Individual and Class Records of Progress

A checklist is an objective score sheet for each health fitness skill taught in the program. By observing and assessing each child's level of performance, you can identify the activities that will assist the child in reaching the performance objective. Use the same checklist to monitor the child's progress during instruction. When the child's performance level changes, you can upgrade the learning tasks (skill components) to the child's new skill level.

To Begin

Decide on one or more health fitness activities to be taught in the program. Become familiar with the description of the performance objective for each activity selected. Review the scoring key on the checklist. Plan assessing activities for the selected skills. The number will depend on the class size, the needs of the children, and the help available to you. Set up testing stations similar to the learning stations. Some teachers use free-play time (after setting up equipment for the objective to be tested) to observe the children.

1. Begin assessing at Skill Level 2 for the particular objective. If the child cannot perform at Skill Level 2, assess for Skill Level 1. If the child demonstrates the skill components for Skill Level 2 (i.e., with modeling, verbal cues, or no cues), the child has achieved functional competence. At the next skill level, Skill Level 3, the child demonstrates maintenance retention of the skill over time.

2. For some children with special needs, you may need to assess their levels of functioning before planning teaching activities. As in step 1, observe and assess the amount and type of assistance (cues) the child needs in descending order (i.e., from verbal cues to total manipulation).

Code	Amount and Type of Assistance
SI	Child initiates demonstrating the skill in the teaching and playing of activities
C	Child demonstrates the skill when given verbal cues with or without demonstration
A	Child demonstrates the skill when given partial assistance or total manipulation throughout the execution of the skill

Record, using the code above, the child's initial assistance level and progress in the comments column of the Class Record of Progress. For some children, this may be the most significant initial progress noted (i.e., from assistance to verbal cues and demonstration).

To Assess

1. Be sure all children are working on objectives at other stations while you are assessing at one station.

2. Make sure enough equipment is available for the skill to be tested.

3. For situps, trunk and leg flexibility, and rest and relaxation skills, have two or three children at the testing station on mats. All can lie on mats and perform skills at the same time. At the end of the trials, record the child's performance on the score sheet.

4. To assess lifting and carrying objects, use a relay. Be sure the starting line and ending line are clearly marked. Divide the children in small groups of two or three. Assess one group or team at a time. At

the end of the trials, record each child's performance on the score sheet.

5. To assess walk-run endurance, have two or three children at the testing station ready to be tested. (The other children in the class should be working at other learning stations.) All children can begin walk-running on the command "go." At the end of the trials, record the child's performance on the score sheet.

6. You may need to modify the assessing activity by using lighter objects to lift and carry, taking the child through the pattern or modeling the activity, or using sign language or an interpreter. Other modifications are an individual structured assessment with no distractions from other children or activities or free play with the equipment. Use mats or movable walls to help cut down on distractions.

To Adapt the Checklists

You can note children's skill components adaptations (i.e., physical devices or other changes) in the comments column on the Class Record of Progress. Other changes can be written under recommendations for individual children or the class. Modifications made for a child can be noted on the Individual Record of Progress. The Class Record of Progress can be adapted for an individual child. Record the name of the child rather than the class, and in the name column, record assessment dates. This adaptation may be needed for children whose progress is erratic, because it provides a base line assessment to find out where to begin teaching and evaluating the child's progress.

The Individual Record of Progress for the end-of-the-year report can be attached to the child's IEP (Individual Education Program) report. The record can also serve as a cumulative record for each child. Such records are very useful for new teachers, substitute teach-ers, aides, and volunteers, as well as parents. The format of the Individual Record of Progress can also be adapted for a Unit Report. The names of all the objectives for a unit—for example, walk-run endurance, running, catching a ball, and rolling a ball—are written rather than the names of the children. Book 8 illustrates the adaptation of the Individual Record of Progress for use in the Home Activities Program and for a Unit Report.

The checklists may be reproduced as needed to implement the play and motor skills program.

CLASS RECORD OF PROGRESS REPORT

CLASS _____ DATE _____

AGE/GRADE _____ TEACHER _____

SCHOOL _____

OBJECTIVE: SITUPS (ABDOMINAL STRENGTH)

SCORING:	SKILL LEVEL 1			SKILL LEVEL 2			SKILL LEVEL 3	PRIMARY RESPONSES:
ASSESSMENT: _____ Date **X** = Achieved **O** = Not Achieved **/** = Partially Achieved REASSESSMENT: _____ Date ⊗ = Achieved Ø = Not Achieved	Three Consecutive Times							N = Not Attending NR = No Response UR = Unrelated Response O = Other (Specify in comments)
NAME	Takes a starting position (lying on back, knees bent 90 degrees, feet flat on mat, arms at sides, feet supported).	Curls up by tucking chin and lifting shoulders (upper back) off the mat.	Returns to starting position in controlled movement by uncurling and lowering head to mat.	Curls up by tucking chin and lifting trunk, completes curl by touching knees with hands.	Returns in controlled manner by uncurling trunk and lowering head to mat, hands on thighs.	Repeats 10 times (or meets standards appropriate for the child).	Two or more play or game activities at home or school demonstrating skill components over six-week period.	COMMENTS
	1	2	3	4	5	6	7	
1.								
2.								
3.								
4.								
5.								
6.								
7.								
8.								
9.								
10.								

Recommendations: Specific changes or conditions in planning for instructions, performance, or diagnostic testing procedures or standards. Please describe what worked best.

_____

_____

_____

_____

_____

_____

CLASS RECORD OF PROGRESS REPORT

CLASS _____   DATE _____

AGE/GRADE _____   TEACHER _____

SCHOOL _____

OBJECTIVE: WALK-RUN FOR ENDURANCE

SCORING:	SKILL LEVEL 1		SKILL LEVEL 2		SKILL LEVEL 3	PRIMARY RESPONSES:
ASSESSMENT: _____Date **X** = Achieved **O** = Not Achieved / = Partially Achieved REASSESSMENT: _____Date ⊗ = Achieved Ø = Not Achieved	Three Consecutive Times					N = Not Attending NR = No Response UR = Unrelated Response O = Other (Specify in comments)
NAME	Walk-runs continuously in any manner at moderate to fast pace for one minute.	Walk-runs continuously in any manner at moderate to fast pace for three minutes.	Walk-runs for two minutes (with two or more periods of nonsupport every ten steps).	Walk-runs for four minutes (with two or more periods of nonsupport every ten steps).	Two or more play or game activities at home or school demonstrating skill components over six-week period.	COMMENTS
	1	2	3	4	5	
1.						
2.						
3.						
4.						
5.						
6.						
7.						
8.						
9.						
10.						

Recommendations: Specific changes or conditions in planning for instructions, performance, or diagnostic testing procedures or standards. Please describe what worked best.

_____

_____

_____

_____

_____

CLASS RECORD OF PROGRESS REPORT

CLASS _____ DATE _____

AGE/GRADE _____ TEACHER _____

SCHOOL _____

OBJECTIVE: TRUNK AND LEG FLEXIBILITY

SCORING:	SKILL LEVEL 1		SKILL LEVEL 2		SKILL LEVEL 3	PRIMARY RESPONSES:
ASSESSMENT: _____ Date **X** = Achieved **O** = Not Achieved **/** = Partially Achieved REASSESSMENT: _____ Date **⊗** = Achieved **Ø** = Not Achieved	Three Consecutive Times					N = Not Attending NR = No Response UR = Unrelated Response O = Other (Specify in comments)
	Takes starting position (sitting on floor, legs straight, feet against sit-and-reach bench or wall), hands on front of thighs.	Bends forward, reaches with hands toward sit-and-reach bench or wall with legs straight, holds for three seconds, and returns to starting position.	Bends forward, reaches with hands toward sit-and-reach bench or wall, holds five seconds, returns to starting position.	Bends forward and touches wall or reaches measurement on sit-and-reach bench established as appropriate for child.	Two or more play or game activities at home or school demonstrating skill components over six-week period.	
NAME	1	2	3	4	5	COMMENTS
1.						
2.						
3.						
4.						
5.						
6.						
7.						
8.						
9.						
10.						

Recommendations: Specific changes or conditions in planning for instructions, performance, or diagnostic testing procedures or standards. Please describe what worked best.

_____

_____

_____

_____

_____

_____

CLASS RECORD OF PROGRESS REPORT

CLASS _____   DATE _____

AGE/GRADE _____   TEACHER _____

SCHOOL _____

OBJECTIVE: LIFT AND CARRY OBJECTS

SCORING:	SKILL LEVEL 1			SKILL LEVEL 2			SKILL LEVEL 3	PRIMARY RESPONSES:
ASSESSMENT:	Three Consecutive Times							N = Not Attending
_____Date	Positions body close to object to be lifted, with weight on both feet, evenly distributed.	Bends knees and lowers body, keeping back straight, and grasps object with both hands.	Lifts object by straightening legs, keeping back straight.	Bends elbows slightly to hold object as close to body as possible in lifting and carrying.	Keeps head, shoulders, and back straight in standing posture alignment.	Carries object with both hands close to body for 10 feet, lowers object to floor in correct manner.	Two or more play or game activities at home or school demonstrating skill components over six-week period.	NR = No Response
X = Achieved								UR = Unrelated Response
O = Not Achieved								O = Other (Specify in comments)
/ = Partially Achieved								
REASSESSMENT:								
_____Date								
⊗ = Achieved								
Ø = Not Achieved								
NAME	1	2	3	4	5	6	7	COMMENTS
1.								
2.								
3.								
4.								
5.								
6.								
7.								
8.								
9.								
10.								

Recommendations: Specific changes or conditions in planning for instructions, performance, or diagnostic testing procedures or standards. Please describe what worked best.

_____

_____

_____

_____

_____

CLASS RECORD OF PROGRESS REPORT

CLASS _____ DATE _____

AGE/GRADE _____ TEACHER _____

SCHOOL _____

OBJECTIVE: REST AND RELAXATION

SCORING:	SKILL LEVEL 1		SKILL LEVEL 2			SKILL LEVEL 3	PRIMARY RESPONSES:
ASSESSMENT: _____Date **X** = Achieved **O** = Not Achieved **/** = Partially Achieved REASSESSMENT: _____Date **Ø** = Achieved **Ø** = Not Achieved	Three Consecutive Times						N = Not Attending NR = No Response UR = Unrelated Response O = Other (Specify in comments)
	Lies on back, arms at sides, legs apart, eyes closed, head turned to left or right (or sits in chair or position appropriate for child).	Recognizes muscular tension in four or more body parts.	Relaxes four or more body parts for one minute beginning with head, face, eyes, and jaw.	Relaxes other body parts until total body is relaxed (breathing, arms, hands, legs, feet, and toes).	Relaxes total body for one minute or more.	Two or more play or game activities at home or school demonstrating skill components over six-week period.	
NAME	1	2	3	4	5	6	COMMENTS
1.							
2.							
3.							
4.							
5.							
6.							
7.							
8.							
9.							
10.							

Recommendations: Specific changes or conditions in planning for instructions, performance, or diagnostic testing procedures or standards. Please describe what worked best.

_____

_____

_____

_____

_____

INDIVIDUAL RECORD OF PROGRESS

Area: Health and Fitness

CHILD: _____

LEVEL: _____

YEAR: _____

TEACHER: _____

SCHOOL: _____

Marking Period	*Date*
Fall Conference (white)	from ____ to ____
Winter Conference (yellow)	from ____ to ____
Spring Conference (pink)	from ____ to ____
End-of-Year (cumulative) Report (blue)	from ____ to ____

Preprimary Play and Motor Skills Activity Program

The Individual Record of Progress lists all of the objectives in which your child receives instruction during the play and motor skills program. The information reported on your child's Individual Record of Progress shows your child's entry performance and progress for a marking period. The end-of-the-year report represents your child's Individual Education Program (IEP) for the objectives selected and taught during the year.

Each objective is broken into small, measurable steps or skill components. This assists the teacher to assess what your child already knew before teaching began and to determine which step to start teaching first. One of the following symbols is marked by each step or skill component of the objective:

X = The child already knew how to perform this step before teaching it began.

O = The child did not know how to perform this step before teaching it began or after instruction of it ended.

Ø = The child did not know how to perform this step before teaching it began, but did learn how to do it during the instruction period.

This information should be helpful to you in planning home activities to strengthen your child's play and motor skills.

Comments

_____

_____

_____

_____

_____

_____

_____

_____

_____

SITUPS (ABDOMINAL STRENGTH)

Date: _____

On an 8-foot mat
Three consecutive times

_____ Takes a starting position (lying on back, knees bent 90 degrees, feet flat on mat, arms at sides, feet supported).

_____ Curls up by tucking chin and lifting shoulders (upper back) off the mat.

_____ Returns to starting position in controlled movement by uncurling and lowering head to mat.

_____ Curls up by tucking chin and lifting trunk, completes curl by touching knees with hand.

_____ Returns in controlled manner by uncurling trunk and lowering head to mat, hands on thighs.

_____ Repeats 10 times (or meet standards appropriate for the child).

_____ Demonstrates above skill in two or more play or game activities at home or school over a six-week period.

WALK-RUN FOR ENDURANCE

Date: _____

Within a clear space of 100 feet
Three consecutive times

_____ Walk-runs continuously in any manner at moderate to fast pace for one minute.

_____ Walk-runs continuously in any manner at moderate to fast pace for three minutes.

_____ Walk-runs for two minutes (with two or more periods of nonsupport every ten steps).

_____ Walk-runs for four minutes (with two or more periods of nonsupport every ten steps).

_____ Demonstrates above skill in two or more play or game activities at home or school over a six-week period.

TRUNK AND LEG FLEXIBILITY

Date: _____

With a sit-and-reach bench or wall
Three consecutive times

_____ Takes starting position (sitting on floor, legs straight, feet against sit-and-reach bench or wall), hands on front of thighs.

_____ Bends forward, reaches with hands toward sit-and-reach bench or wall with legs straight, holds for three seconds, and returns to starting position.

_____ Bends forward, reaches with hands toward sit-and-reach bench or wall, holds five seconds, returns to starting position.

_____ Bends forward and touches wall or reaches measurement on sit-and-reach bench established as appropriate for child.

_____ Demonstrates above skill in two or more play or game activities at home or school over a six-week period.

LIFT AND CARRY OBJECTS

Date: _____

Within a space of 10 feet
Three consecutive times

_____ Positions body close to object to be lifted, with weight on both feet, evenly distributed.

_____ Bends knees and lowers body, keeping back straight, and grasps object with both hands.

_____ Lifts object by straightening legs, keeping back straight.

_____ Bends elbows slightly to hold object as close to body as possible in lifting and carrying.

_____ Keeps head, shoulders, and back straight in standing posture alignment.

_____ Carries object with both hands close to body for 10 feet, lowers object in correct manner.

_____ Demonstrates above skill in two or more play or game activities at home or school over a six-week period.

REST AND RELAXATION

Date: _____

On an 8-foot mat in quiet-time space
Three consecutive times

_____ Lies on back, arms at sides, legs apart, eyes closed, head turned to left or right (or sits in chair or position appropriate for child).

_____ Recognizes muscular tension in four or more body parts (head turning from side to side, eyes squeezed closed, lips tight, jaw clenched, breathing fast or holding breath, arms turned in or moving, fist clenched or fingers moving, foot rigid or moving, toes curled or rigid).

_____ Relaxes four or more body parts for one minute, beginning with head, face, eyes, and jaw.

_____ Relaxes other body parts until total body is relaxed (breathing, arms, hands, legs, feet, and toes).

_____ Relaxes total body for one minute or more.

_____ Demonstrates above skill in two or more play or game activities at home or school over a six-week period.

Games

Game Selection

The following game sheets will help you select and plan game activities. They include the names of the games in alphabetical order, formation, directions, equipment, locomotor skills, and type of play activity. Consider the following points when selecting games:

1. Skills and objectives of your program

2. Interest of the child

3. Equipment and rules

4. Adaptability of physical difficulty level in order to match each child's ability

5. Activity for healthy growth and development

6. Social play skill development, such as taking turns, sharing equipment, playing with others, and following and leading

Games can foster creativity. Children enjoy making up, interpreting, and creating their own activities, whether playing alone, with a partner, or with a small group. The time you take to provide opportunities for each child to explore and create will be well spent. One further note. Children can easily create or adapt games matched to their mobility, even if limited by crutches, braces, or wheelchairs. Health fitness activities involve moving from here to there. These children easily comprehend how to get to "there" with their own expertise for movement.

Following are some suggestions for adapting the physical difficulty level of games and a sequential list of social play development:

Adapting Games

To Change	Use	Example
1. Boundaries	Larger or smaller space	Change play space size (width, length).
2. Equipment	Larger or smaller sizes, weights, or heights, or specially adapted equipment for some children (such as guide-rails, inclines rather than stairs, brightly colored mats)	Lift different objects, such as medicine ball.
3. Rules	More or fewer rules	In Shuttle Run Relay, have children walk first or continue running.

To Change	Use	Example
4. Actions	More or fewer actions to be performed at one time; play in stationary positions, using various body parts	Change number of times action is repeated, or begin with one position only (starting position).
5. Time of play	Longer or shorter time; frequent rest periods	In Lift and Pass, pass for 5 seconds, then 10 seconds.

To adapt games to other special needs, you might also use buddies and spotters, sign language gestures, or place the child near leader.

Sequential Development of Social Play

Sequence	Description	Example of Play Activity
Individual Play	Child plays alone and independently with toys that are different from those used by other children within speaking distance.	Child plays in assigned area, lifting and carrying object. Other children are playing with same objects nearby.
Parallel Play	Child plays independently beside, rather than with, other children.	Child plays with boxes to lift and carry. Does situps, walk-runs. Other children have objects to lift, do situps or sit-reach. No interaction between children.
Associate Play	Child plays with other children. There is interaction between children, but there are no common goals.	Child plays with other children lifting and carrying objects, doing situps or sit-reach. Children play as partners or follow the leader.
Cooperative Play	Child plays within a group organized for playing formal games. Group is goal directed.	Children play games together as team, doing activities that involve lifting and carrying objects, walk-run activities, resting and relaxing.

Game Sheet Lesson Plans

Games	Organization	Description/Instructions	Equipment	Skills	Type of Play Activity
Figure 8 Run	start ✗✗✗✗ (figure 8 diagram)	Children line up behind start. Run around the figure 8 until whistle blows.	Taped figure 8; whistle	Walk-run for endurance	Individual, partners, small group, large group
Follow the Leader	Line ++++++ Circle (diagram with leader T)	Teacher leads children in some situps, leg lifts, run-walk, lifting objects. Then a child becomes new leader.	Mats, boxes, cones	All health fitness skills	Small group, large group
Giants and Dwarfs	Scatter or circle (X marks scattered)	Children stand in circle or stand scattered around room. Teach them the words: "Let us be little or small, and then let us stand up straight and tall. We'll be giants one and all." Have children imitate action words. Emphasize bending and stretching trunk and legs.	None	Trunk and leg flexibility	Partners, small group, large group

Book 4: Health Fitness Activities   57

GAME SHEET LESSON PLANS

GAMES	ORGANIZATION	DESCRIPTION/INSTRUCTIONS	EQUIPMENT	SKILLS	TYPE OF PLAY ACTIVITY
I Am a Balloon	Scatter X X X X X X X X	Ask children to shake as loosely and floppily as possible. Say, "You are a saggy balloon, and you have no air in you. Can you go limp? When you hear 'shhh,' you are being slowly filled with air. Are you as big as you can be? Full? Tight? Oh! You have a slow leak—psss. You are beginning to collapse and go limp."	None	Relaxation	Individual, partners, small group, large group
Jello Jiggle	Scatter X X X X X X X X	Ask children to find a spot on the floor. Ask if they've ever seen a bowl of jello jiggle. "Let your arms, shoulders, head, wobble. Can you wiggle with a friend? Make up a dance, 'Juggle Jiggle.'"	None	Relaxation	Individual, partners, small group, large group
Let's Relax	Scatter X X X X X X X X	Have children lie on their backs with eyes closed, arms away from body. Tell them, "Lie still. Don't move, keep eyes closed. Relax." Have them tense and relax various body parts. "Make a fist. Hold tight, let it go." Use calm voice, soft music, dim lights.	Mats	Relaxation	Individual partners, small group, large group

GAME SHEET LESSON PLANS

GAMES	ORGANIZATION	DESCRIPTION/INSTRUCTIONS	EQUIPMENT	SKILLS	TYPE OF PLAY ACTIVITY
Lift a Box	Lines XXXXXXX A XXXXXXX B	Give each child a number. Tell them which box, A or B, is theirs. "When I call your number, you must run to box and lift it. Hand it to the teacher and run back to your place. First person who gets back to spot scores a point for that team."	Two 10-lb. boxes	Lift and carry	Teams; small group, large group
Lift and Pass	Circle X X X X X X X X X X	Children form a circle. Place blocks and balls in center. Select one child to begin. Have child choose a ball or block from floor, lift it up, pass it to child on right. Have object passed completely around the circle. Continue with other objects of different weights.	Balls, blocks of various sizes	Lift and carry	Small group, large group
Lifting Relay	Line table boxes ☐ ☐ ☐ XXX XXX XXX	Divide children into teams. One from each team walks or runs to boxes, lifts a box and carries it to the table, then runs back and tags next child to take turn.	Table; one box per team	Lift and carry	Teams; small group, large group

Game Sheet Lesson Plans

Games	Organization	Description/Instructions	Equipment	Skills	Type of Play Activity
Line Carry	Line ↑↑↑↑↑ × × × × × red line	Give each child an object to carry. On cue, all begin walking across the room. Say, "Carry your object to the red line. Carry it back." Can give awards to first, second, third. Can do as a partner relay (carry it down, other carries it back).	Objects to carry (toys, books)	Lift and carry	Relay; partners, small group, large group
Magic Ball	Circle × × × × × × × × × ×	Children sit in circle on carpet squares. Pass ball around circle and say verse: "The Magic Ball goes around and round. If you're the one to touch it last, then for you the game is past. You're out." On word "out," child must leave circle for one turn.	Nerf ball; carpet squares	Lift and carry	Small group, large group
Medicine Ball	Line × × × → 乇 × × × → 乇	Children lift and carry a medicine ball to the chair and back again. Lines race with each other.	Medicine balls; chairs	Lift and carry	Relay; small group, large group

Game Sheet Lesson Plans

Games	Organization	Description/Instructions	Equipment	Skills	Type of Play Activity
Moving Game	Scatter X X X X X X	Have children move building blocks from one area to another. Encourage them to use various ways to transport building materials (wagons, trucks). Can vary by lifting and stacking boxes to build a house or cave.	Small trucks; wagons; blocks or boxes	Lift and carry	Individual, partners, small group, large group
Obstacle Course	Line x x x ☐ Station 1 ☐ Station 2 ☐ Station 3	When first child completes second station, next child begins.	Mats, boxes, cones	All health fitness skills	Individual, partners, small group, large group
Raggedy Ann and Andy	Scatter X X X X X	Have children be Raggedy Ann or Andy filled with straw. They dance and play until they start losing straw. Then they collapse. When they are filled up with straw again, they can run and play again. Stress relaxation of the body.	None	Relaxation	Individual, partners, small group, large group

Book 4: Health Fitness Activities   61

Game Sheet Lesson Plans

Games	Organization	Description/Instructions	Equipment	Skills	Type of Play Activity
Scatter Play	Scatter X X X X X X X X	Scatter one object per person around the room. Say, "Find an object to hold. Lift and hold the object when music begins. Walk, carrying object. When music stops, put object down and find another one to carry."	One object per person (vary sizes)	Lift and carry	Individual, partners, small group, large group
Shuttle Run Relay	Line XXX ⇵ XXX ⇵ wall	Have 2 to 4 children in each line. Tell them to stand behind the line. "Run to the wall. Jump and touch as high as you can. Go back to start. Then next child goes." Can use stop watch.	Taped lines; wall	Trunk and leg flexibility	Partners, small group, large group
Simon Says	Circle x T x x x x x x x	One child or teacher is leader. All must perform skill if he or she says, "Simon says do this." If just "do this," children must not do the skill.	None	All health fitness skills	Partners, small group, large group